THE CAREGIVER

Helping You and Your Patient Through the Dementia Journey

Thomas M. Garasic

ISBN 979-8-89485-298-0 (Paperback)
ISBN 979-8-89485-299-7 (Digital)

Covenant Books
11661 Hwy 707
Murrells Inlet, SC 29576
www.covenantbooks.com

INTRODUCTION

I dedicate this information to my wife of fifty-five years, Martha Irene Garasic, who was a private educator and who taught me through her actions how to care for her during her journey with dementia. It is my deepest desire to honor her and to help others benefit from our family's experiences.

I learned how to best assist my wife with help from ProMedica's Arden Courts webinars conducted by Dr. Tam Cummings, along with St. Barnabas's Marjorie Hobaugh and Anna Foust. Invaluable information was also gleaned from the Alzheimer's Association, in conjunction with counseling, care and consultation by Dr. John Wisneski from UPMC and with Dr. Jagan Pillai from the Cleveland Clinic.

I have learned and experienced many things during the five years I've spent caring for my wife. I am not a doctor, and my objective is not to give medical advice. My intention here, instead, is to provide effective, practical strategies for handling potential challenges as the caregiver for someone with dementia. My goal in writing this manual is to provide help for anyone in caring for a loved one while not neglecting themselves. Ultimately, dementia is a family journey. And although each phase is unique, there are also common elements. Ultimately, I hope that my experiences will help dementia families navigate the challenges and process of this cruel disease with greater clarity and confidence!

L—living

I—in

F—forgetful

E—environments

This manual provides space in each section for your personal notes about a specific task or dates when you have accomplished that task. You will, at times, be overwhelmed by the care you need to administer. Your notes will assure you that you have initiated and completed the task. Personal notes will give you confidence that you are doing a "great job" in your caregiving. There should be no more "would've," "could've," or "should've" statements involved in any aspect of caring for a patient with dementia. As a caregiver, you must do the job to the best of your ability! Some people may suggest that "dementia caregiving" is a journey. Rather, it is actually "uncharted territory." So plan to put on your work boots and wade right in. It is "muddy" out there.

LET'S GET STARTED

Create three folders: A medical folder, a financial folder, and a legal folder.

The Medical Folder

This consists of the primary care physician's (PCP) name and all the phone numbers needed to contact that doctor including who they may use to cover when they are not available. Include the same information regarding the neurologist involved in the case.

Caregivers. If you are using caregivers, you may want to also include all of the contact information for the people involved with your dementia patient, including night numbers.

Powers of attorney (POAs) for your patient. You should also have a designated POA for yourself in case of an unexpected emergency. You *never know what might occur in the future.*

Medical personnel who come to your house. Include the names and providing organizations, along with phone numbers and evening contacts, for all medical personnel who are connected with your patient.

Palliative care information. This is usually available through your PCP. Make sure the doctor explains what palliative care entails. Make sure that you understand when you may need this care and how to go about obtaining it.

Hospice care information. This is also available through your PCP. Know how to procure the services when they are needed. (This is very important!)

All medications that are to be taken each day. Note which meds are taken in the AM and which are to be taken in the PM. Also create a list specifying when they were started and the dosage of each med, which will be listed on the bottle. Keep an updated list of all medications in an accessible and visible place in each car that may be driven with the patient; in the event of an accident, those medications may be critical to the care of the patient.

This folder will probably become *very large* in order to include all of the information that you may need. *Note: It's important to date everything in this folder.*

Begin by listing the changes in the patient's actions. Include information such as "Unable to get out of bed without help" or "Dominant side having movement problems" or "Handshakes" or "Unable to get out of chair by himself," etc.

List all changes as they occur, along with relevant dates, and bring that list with you to the doctor's office so that he/she can begin to evaluate the patient's progress. It is probably unrealistic to proceed to the doctor's office believing that you will be able to remember everything which has occurred. However, with the proper organization, you should be able to provide accurate information and will not be wasting valuable time at the office visit. Again, always remember to create the list and to take it with you!

You will also need to make sure you have all relevant appointments noted on a master calendar. Note that you may always need to make a special effort to arrive on time. However, be aware that this may become an increasing challenge as the patient's dementia progresses! Plan the time necessary to prepare departure to be on time for all appointments.

The Financial Folder

This folder includes information about your financial advisor and should list all accounts—both joint and individual. These might be investments, all retirement accounts, Social Security information, saving accounts, checking accounts, credit card accounts and all insurance including life insurance and health insurance. Include names, account numbers, and phone numbers of financial institutions. Make sure you are up-to-date on all this information. Question everyone and everything on each of these accounts. You do not need to let the bankers know the person you are caring for has dementia. Let them know you are the POA and are just updating all the information for your records. The bankers are on a "need to know basis," and you do not need to provide them with any additional and unnecessary information.

Make sure you maintain at least one account with both of your names on it. You may need it for that one time that a check arrives and says both of your names with an *and* between them. The bank will be unable to process the financial instrument without having that account open.

The Legal Folder

Lawyers can assist you with the POAs, last will and testament, and living will. Make sure you have all the contact information for the lawyer including phone numbers, addresses, and other contacts when they may not be available. Do this in the beginning stages of the disease so the patient can be helpful in furnishing you and the lawyer with information for an accurate legal document. Make copies of the POA because when you show up to most health care facilities, their personnel may not provide information willingly, and the POA will move that process along quickly and legally. You will need those POAs for the financial advisor and for changing information on life insurance policies and other legal documents and instruments. You will be amazed at how often they are required just to move forward with simple requests.

Notes:

TYPES OF DEMENTIA

Dementia is an "umbrella term" that says this person is at a stage when, because of their memory/judgment/language/or broadly thinking problems, they cannot take care of themselves independently. You really need to know what the cause of dementia is in the person you are caring for has and how it is affecting them. As dementia does not happen overnight, we know that in the years before the stage of dementia, the person is usually having changes in memory/judgment/language or thinking. However, by compensating, they are still able to care for themselves at home independently. This stage is called mild cognitive impairment (MCI). There are again different causes or reasons for getting MCI stage; they also include Alzheimer's disease, FTD, Lewy body, Parkinson etc. There are tests your physician can run to help diagnose the underlying cause of MCI or dementia. Understanding the cause of dementia is critical information to help target the treatment and management of your loved one over this stage of life when they might be in your day-to-day care.

Dementia is not one-size-fits-all in terms of manifestation and treatment. There are nine common types of dementia:

1. Alzheimer's disease is a progressive brain disease that involves the parts of the brain that control thoughts, memory, and language.

2. Lewy body dementia is the result of abnormal deposits of protein in the brain. The effects lead to problems with thinking, movement, behavior, and mood.

3. Frontotemporal dementia (FTD) is the result of damage to neurons in the frontal and temporal lobes of the brain. This causes unusual behaviors, emotional problems, trouble communicating, and difficulty walking.

4. Vascular dementia is brain damage caused by multiple strokes, high cholesterol, diabetes, and problems with heartbeat rhythm.

5. Parkinson's disease dementia causes uncontrollable tremors or swaying, slowed movement, impaired posture and balance, and changes in speech and voice.

6. Wernicke-Korsakoff syndrome is a brain condition associated with alcohol abuse.

7. Huntington's dementia is an inherited condition in which nerve cells in the brain break down over time.

8. Chronic traumatic encephalopathy (CTE) is the result of chronic traumatic injury such as repeated head injury and blows to the head.

9. Mixed dementia is a combination of conditions resulted in a mixture of symptoms.

You really need to know which form of dementia the person that you are caring for has and how it is affecting them. Get all of the testing done. Your thinking process is that you are no longer the husband, wife, daughter, or son. At this point, you have become "the caregiver." This is your new job. It may come without pay or recognition. However, you do bring to this job a sense of commitment, love, fulfillment, confidence, and knowledge about your patient. More importantly, you get to put all of that to work.

Continue to work closely with your doctors to keep both you and the patient comfortable. Doctors may start with the written test, but you still need an MRI, CAT scan, blood draw, and spinal tap to determine the specific form of dementia. Your neurologist will be able help you throughout the process of engaging in all of the testing. You need to know what is going on in the brain and what is coming back from the brain so you know what is staying in the brain. This will tell you what disease is destroying which part of the brain as this will give you the information needed on how to begin treating the patient. Don't let your health insurance company talk you out of the testing.

Just remember that you are the one caring for your patient, and it's unlikely that anyone from your insurance company will be there to help you navigate the process.

DEMENTIA STAGES

Stage 1. No visible cognitive decline and generally no apparent or recognizable changes in the patient.

Stage 2. Very mild cognitive impairment. Most doctors do not recognize dementia at this stage. Most individuals exhibit denial or avoidance of the topic at this time and associate it with age.

Stage 3. Increasing levels of impairment. Again, doctors and many people relate this impairment to age (you're just older).

Stage 4. Mild dementia with moderate decline. Decreased knowledge of recent events but still recognizing people and places.

Stage 5. Moderate dementia and moderate impairment. The patient needs assistance to live day-to-day. Patients have trouble recalling major events and become disoriented regarding time and place. Incontinence may begin to become an issue.

Stage 6. Severe cognitive impairment becomes noticeable. The patient requires assistance in movements and does not recognize the spouse or sometimes his or her children. They need help to survive day-to-day. They have a loss of willpower due to the loss of thought processes. Incontinence becomes an issue.

Stage 7. Very severe cognitive impairment. They have loss of speech and are dependent on the caregiver for survival. The end is Near.

In retrospect, these are the stages that I noticed in my wife as she moved through the first three stages; no one noticed. However, I began to see changes in her movements and actions. The remaining stages were my experiences as she went through each stage and the diminishing effect it had on her. Again, I am not a doctor. I am just sharing what I experienced with my wife from her initial symptoms to her diagnosis and eventual passing away.

As dementia progresses, friends, family, and phone calls disappear because most people do not know how to talk to or interact with dementia patients. Life becomes lonely because it's just you and the dementia patient each day. This is where humor and a bit of "acting" are needed for both of you to enjoy the time you have remaining together. It's important to try to make your daily life together as satisfying as possible!

Once your patient begins to speak, try to listen to him or her with careful attention. These conversations will begin to tell you "where they are mentally" as well as "in what time frame they seem to be thinking." Dementia patients are somewhat like "time travelers." They may seem to be in the 1970s at times, move into the '80s, and occasionally may appear to be fully in the present.

On occasion, a dementia patient may also want to speak with someone from their past or someone that's been deceased for a long time. They may say something like "Mom lives just across the street so let's stop and visit her" when Mom passed away many years before. Your answer might be that "Mom has a doctor's appointment and won't be home for visitors." You may be making up story after story, but don't stop paying attention to their comments, conversations, or verbiage because these will help you relate to them when you try to communicate.

You now need to become an "actor" of sorts. You can begin to fill in the time so they can relate to the conversation. You may even have to make up stories about people, places, or events. But these stories will help to calm the dementia patient down if they can relate to them. Frequently, these patients may become agitated whenever they are frustrated and cannot understand what is going on or they are not understanding the conversation. Only speak to a dementia patient face-to-face; speak softly, and never raise your voice.

However, *do not* talk about them or their dementia to anyone while they are with you or can hear you speaking. This would most likely be frustrating for them because they are unable to respond in the time frame of your conversation. It will begin to take longer for them to respond to questions or comments because their brain is not working at full capacity. You need sufficient patience to ask questions and then wait for an answer, which could require up to fifteen seconds! Standing there and waiting for that amount of time may prove to be very uncomfortable for both of you. Please exercise patience!

Notes:

Anatomy and Functional Areas of the Brain

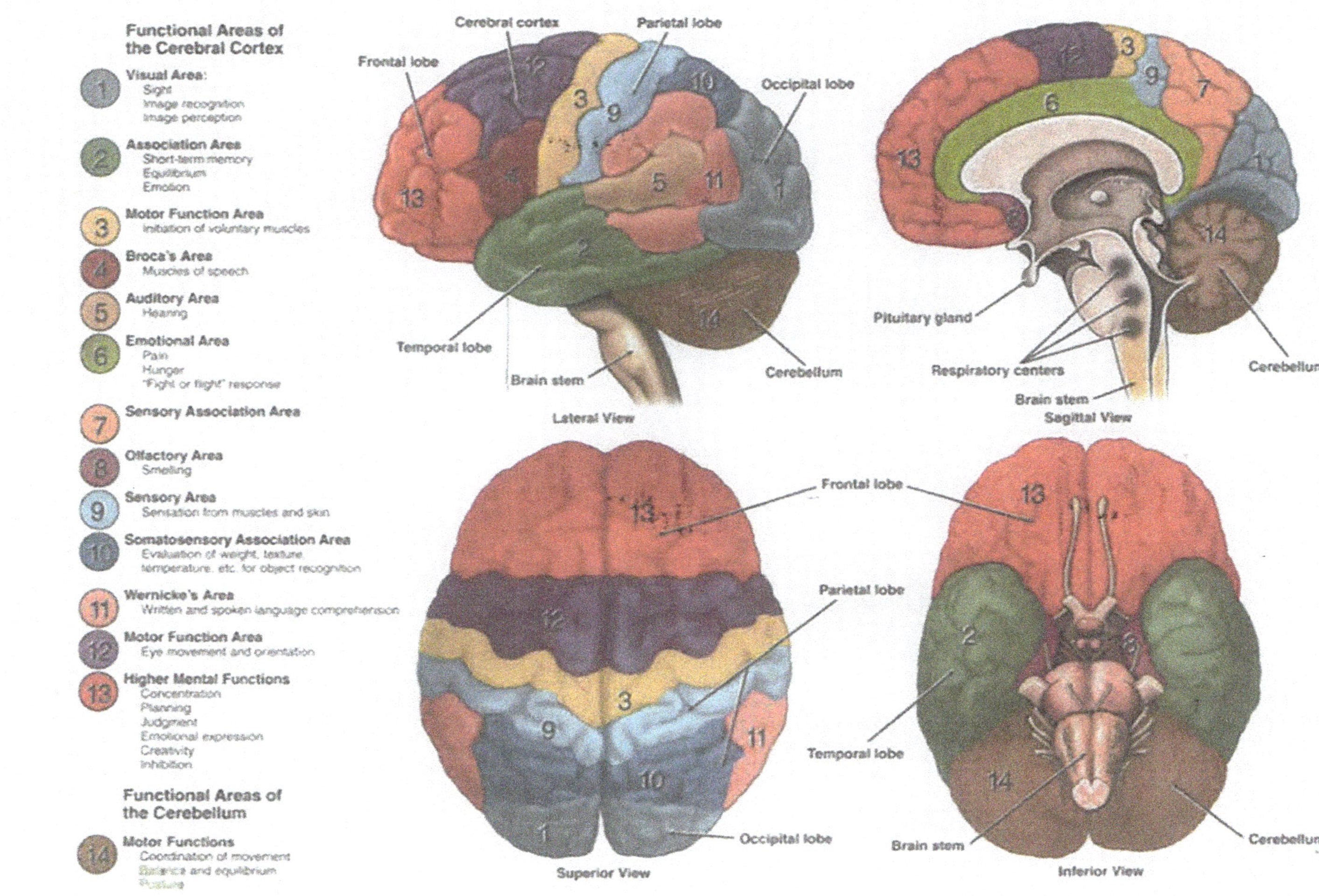

THE FAMILY MEETING

You need to schedule this meeting, but you *must* have an agenda since you are caring for the patient. Make sure you have an idea of who can help with what, a list of chores to be allocated, and how often each family member is expected to be involved. Note that you may have to negotiate time and tasks, but this should give you a starting point. Critical areas of need are the following:

- Meals
- Financial help
- Food purchasing
- Yard work
- Housework

Create a schedule for tasks and identify individuals responsible for each so you have time to take care of the patient and yourself.

The most salient feature here is to let the family know that because of stress, anxiety, and 24/7 care, three out of ten caregivers pass away before the patient they are caring for does. You want to make sure that this does not happen to you. Family members will most likely understand the significance of this because caregiving then becomes their task.

Example: Having a patient's son cut grass and trim bushes once a week on Saturday mornings while daughter number 1 helps clean the house on Thursday evenings and daughter number 2 shops for food on Wednesday mornings. Make a list for the children or other family members that are helping.

Notes:

THE CHILDREN

Single Family

If you've had children together, let them *help*. They are not your counselors or managers. You are the director. You tell them what you need. Children can help with finances, or they can help with watching the patient while you are shopping, or you can send them shopping for food and household items.

If you need help financially, ask them to purchase those food and household items for mom or dad. If they do not get the hints, let them know it's their contribution to the effort of caring for mom or dad. Be nice about it but also remain firm!

You are there 24/7 while they most likely only come by when it's convenient for them. But do not get into a verbal confrontation because no one will probably win and other unexpected personal issues may arise.

Our family worked well together. The children were located in Florida, California, and locally. They were all very enthusiastic about spending time with their mom, both by themselves as well as along with their families. I believe that helps both the patient and children in the dementia process.

Blended Families

For obvious reasons, these may tend to be somewhat more difficult to negotiate or navigate. Every child may have a different concept or alternate suggestion on how best to care for mom or dad.

They may each be also reluctant at some level to "pitch in." No one may wish to do the actual work necessary, but individually, each may have "all" the answers. Let them know that *you* are running the show, and you need all of their support. Tell them, "I shall request help from each of you as it is needed!" It is also imperative that this request be brought up at the initial family meeting.

Make a list of all people who should be helping and what they are going to do to help you. But it's important to be concrete! Be sure to include the times and dates of what they are committing to do along with the frequency of expected visits. Make detailed notes so you can refresh their memories if they forget, which is to be expected.

Notes:

PREPARING THE HOUSE FOR THE PATIENT

Your house is your "home and castle" which you have lovingly decorated and beautifully appointed. However, for a patient with dementia, a room filled with numerous appointments and decorations may also become a hazard and a pitfall.

Begin the "redecorating and rearranging process" with those areas where the patient is having the most trouble. If getting out of bed becomes an issue, consider removing the bed frames, which are usually eight to ten inches high. At this point, the box spring/foundation set and mattress will then be on the floor. This should allow the patient's feet to easily touch the floor. But always make sure their hips and knees are in line when they arise for ease in getting out of bed!

Keep in mind that if their hips are below their knees, the patient will have problems getting out of bed or a chair without assistance. Dementia patients usually want to have their feet touch the floor before they get up. Most likely that contributes to feelings of security and stability. In addition, they may find it easier to get up on their own with the lower bed.

The patient will begin to need bed pads and undergarments at some point, so be prepared to purchase them. There are also companies that will ship pads and undergarments to you on a scheduled basis, and these should also be much less expensive than the same items purchased at a drug store. This service may prove to be the most convenient and could potentially save you money. I used a company called *Unique Wellness*. They can be reached at 1-888-936-7770. This company performed like clockwork, consistently shipping me supplies every three weeks, as scheduled.

There may also be items around the house that you need to remove because they may cause harm to the patient. For example, a decorative bowl of wax fruit may need to be removed because the patient may believe that it is real fruit and attempt to eat it. If you need to have candles lit in your home, use battery-operated candles instead. The patient may wish to light candles in the middle of the night while people are sleeping. Potentially, that could cause a fire, which may prove to be catastrophic. If they light candles, you can no longer scold them; just remove the candles and the lighter. The paradigm has shifted.

Also try to anticipate other potential problems as you move throughout your home and correct them immediately as you might with a toddler! Block stairways so the patient will not be at risk to inadvertently fall down a set of stairs. Using child gates placed at chest level should help.

Throw rugs should also be removed. However, you may wish to do this while the patient is sleeping to avoid creating an issue with them saying something like "That was my favorite carpet! Why are you throwing it away?"

Remove all tripping hazards and, if possible, install grab bars in all areas that have a single step which leads into another room. This should help to prevent inadvertent tripping and make it easier and safer for the patient to get around. It is best to do this as soon as possible so you do not forget to do so at a future time!

To help prevent any cooking issues, you may need to announce to the patient in your best acting mode that you have become "their personal chef "and will be at their service for all meals.

If the stove becomes a problem because the patient insists on helping with meal preparation, you may have to remove the knobs from the burner and oven and store them in a cabinet so that the patient does not arbitrarily or inadvertently turn them on and off.

The dishwasher can also become a hazard for some patients. These individuals may or may not wash all the dishes from a complete dinner service. However, sometimes, he or she may start the dishwasher with just a single dish in it and push the button for a three-hour wash cycle, to little purpose.

To prevent this unnecessary use of soap, water, and energy, simply hide the soap pellets in an area where the patient will not expect to find them. When that happens, there is a good chance that they will no longer turn the dishwasher on, and that problem will be solved.

And before using the dishwasher, always look inside it first because you never know what items they may have placed inside such as shoes, clothing, car keys, mail, or trash. Obviously, you don't wish to cause a properly functioning dishwasher to have unnecessary problems!

The refrigerator is normally a repository for little more than food and beverages. But it may also hide other things that some patients unknowingly place there. These might include keys, trash, clothing, and anything that the patient may have been walking around holding during the day. And if the dementia patient routinely begins to retrieve and start eating raw food that should be cooked, you may need to place a lock on your refrigerator door.

Sharp kitchen items such as knives, scissors, and other sharp objects need to be placed in a drawer or cabinet that the patient will not be able to find. This is for your protection as well as theirs.

But a word of caution here. If you believe that blocking off the kitchen entrance will eliminate that danger, be aware that the patient will most likely augment the situation by finding another means to enter, sometimes over the counter or under the chairs.

Naturally, you are doing this for the patient's protection, but he or she may not actually realize that. Again, you cannot scold them about mistakes because patients usually have no idea that they are making mistakes. Your job is to solve the problem at hand and speak softly to them even if you are upset. You need to get a grip on your new outlook so it will help both of you to do well.

Start by speaking *softly* as often as possible no matter what is happening. If you need the patient to do something specific, whispering becomes the best method to get them to believe it is their idea. That concept worked for me. It's worth a try for you.

If, by chance, the patient helps you in the kitchen with chores, you need to pay attention to every movement. Dropped plates and glasses may cause serious injuries, so you need to move the patient away from the accident quickly and in a calm voice so they will respond to your direction. I cannot stress enough how important it is to pay attention to every movement and action and to respond accordingly and in a calm manner!

Also, find a recent picture of your patient and take it to your local police department. Explain to them that your patient suffers from dementia and that if a law enforcement officer sees him or her walking around alone in an attire which is inappropriate for the season, the patient should be returned to a specific address. You may find the police may begin patrolling your area a little more often, which certainly isn't a bad thing!

Call 911 and ask for a supervisor to explain your situation in caring for your patient. If something happens to you and you need to call 911, give the supervisor all the information on how to get access into your house to assist you.

Indicate where you hide the key and the alarm code if you have a security system. If you have a pet, they should also be made aware of that and any other pertinent information that may help them to enter your home safely and easily.

And make sure to let them know that the patient may be unable to assist or help in any way. But provide phone numbers to have someone arrive at your house to care for your patient. Make sure you let your support people know that they are on such a list with 911 for assistance in case of an emergency. You generally will need to get their approval before you give their names and phone numbers to the 911 supervisor.

You most likely will also need to give the supervisor the names and phone numbers of three support people so that, upon arrival, the ambulance can take care of you. Be sure to let these people know that they are on the 911 list and may get a call from someone that may be coming to your house to take care of you in an emergency. Make sure they willingly agree to do this and are not just saying yes to be agreeable. Ask them whether they will be willing to answer the phone calls even if the phone rings and the emergency occurs in the middle of the night.

Notes:

(Names and phone numbers)

Dates and times you talked to the police and the officer's name

Date and time you talked to 911 and the supervisor's name

Include any other information you feel necessary to note.

PERSONAL HYGIENE

You can make personal hygiene and bath time sound inviting by calling it *spa time*. Set up a routine and do the same actions in the same order *every day*. If you wake the patient, be consistent; set the alarm for the same time every single day. As part of the wake up routine, tell them your name and indicate that you're the favorite person in their life. Mention the time, date, and year. Ham it up! Make the conversation consistent every day and, if possible, wear the same outfit so that they begin to recognize you as the person waking them up. You may need two or three sets of the same outfits to do this task, but consistency is the key to keeping them comfortable and calm because they know what to expect from you at that time.

In the bathroom, you may need to have a support bar installed on the commode. Try installing the bar only on the patient dominate side with the support arm because it will become easier to wipe the patient after usage. If two support arms are installed, you will have trouble with spreading their legs to wipe them clean. Give them a chance to perform the task, but if they become unable, then you must become the person to take over. "You did hear me say it's muddy out there."

You really need a walk-in shower to work with your patients. The tub is next to impossible for either of you in trying to bathe the patient. The bathroom floor color and shower floor color need to be very similar because the patient may feel that they are stepping into a hole if the colors are radically different. And because they do not want to fall, they become very difficult to get into the shower.

If you need to make the shower floor color the same as the bathroom floor color than go to Home Depot and purchase a mat that is similar to the color of the bathroom floor; this will help solve the problem. Your shower will also need to have a handrail and bars to support the patient along with a shower seat. If they stand up, keep the shower seat hidden until it is absolutely necessary. Wash the patient the same way each time; again, consistency is the key. If they have an accident in the shower, clean it up, and move on. Remember in the beginning I said, "It is muddy out there," so get over it, no scolding.

When giving the patient medications, make sure they swallow all pills. The best way to make sure they swallowed the pills is to then brush their teeth because you will have their mouth open to also see if the meds are gone. This tip is most helpful because they sometimes hold the med in their mouth and then spit them out in a glass of water or coffee or whatever they are drinking next. They are beginning to lose their taste sensation so even though the medication would taste terrible in their mouth, they are unable to taste the meds.

When you begin the dressing process, make sure you comb the hair. If the patient is female, place some makeup on her and make her look great and complement her. Remember, you are becoming the actor playing the role of caretaker. This makes the process easier for all. It's "showtime."

Dress the patient for the day. Make sure clothes are comfortable and easy to get off and on. You may put them in shorts all year long if they are not going out. Purchase clothes that go on easy and go off easy. Zippers, elastic waists, and loose pullovers are good, but stay clear of buttons. The buttons are sometimes found in the mouth and are a choking hazard. If finances are tight, go to secondhand or consignment shops where prices are very good. Do not be embarrassed to go to those shops since your patient may only wear clothing once or twice and soil the articles so badly that you need to throw everything away.

You may also take your patient's clothes, those that they cannot wear any longer, to the consignment shop to sell and be able to bring your cost down and lighten your load financially. Consignment shops often have programs that can sometimes help you when clothes are there for a long period. They sometimes donate them, and you may end up the recipient of this good fortune. Talk to the owners about your caregiving, and they will help, I'm sure.

Select shoes for your patient that best fits the situation. If they are staying in all day, you may not need to put shoes on them at all. Walking barefoot is quite comfortable, and they may seem surer of their steps. There are support socks with gripper bottoms that are also good because they keep pressure on your patient's legs and gives them sure footing. Sometimes, that sure footing becomes a drag in carpeted rooms and may cause problems. Again, pay attention to anything new that you try and make sure it works in the patient's best interest. You may use sandals or comfortable shoes when going out depending on the season. Remember, they cannot really tell you if they are too warm or too cold, so watch their actions. It is easier to take off the jacket than to wish you had put one on, and the same goes for hats, gloves, and scarfs.

Notes:

MIRROR, MIRROR ON THE WALL

If your patient is talking about past events from the seventies or eighties, you may need to redirect their view in the mirror because they will not recognize the person that they are seeing. Redirecting may involve just getting in front of them and turning them around so they see you and not the mirror. The person that they see may confuse them because they do not recognize themselves. Just say nothing, and move on or shrug your shoulders. You really do not need to explain everything all the time.

Notes:

OUTSIDE SPACES

Have a designated outside space where you take your patient. Use this space as a room to get fresh air, sunshine, and a different view. It is relaxing, but if your outside space is a deck, there may be spaces between floor boards that the patient may be afraid of falling through, so you may have a problem getting them on the patio. Get a sample carpet runner from the door to their chair because the fear of their falling through holes then goes away. They may sit in that chair on their own. If you have a special place for them to sit, place a glass of water or their favorite beverage or cookies or candy on the table in front of their chair so they will feel like a special treat is there for them and become comfortable with the seating arrangement.

You may also be consistent engaging in this routine at the same time every day since consistency is the key to success. If the special seating takes place outdoors, have a plan B in place for in case it rains. This break is also good for the caregiver since it pauses the day's activities. Remember: *Do not leave the patient alone.* You never know what unexpected movement they will make on the spur of the moment. The patient may decide to walk off, fall over the railing, etc. If you place them in a passive restraint chair, that is a chair that has the hips below the knees, they will have a much harder time getting out, and you may have to help them (lifting picture on next page).

The Adirondack chair is a prime example of passive seating. You may need cushions if your person is sitting in one of those types because they are either wood or plastic and not very soft.

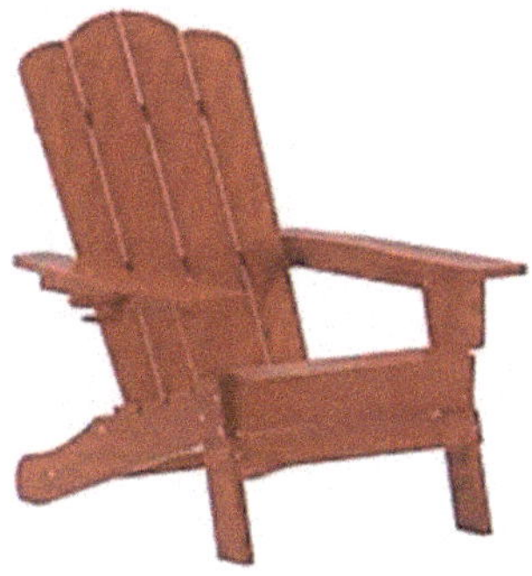

Notes:

LIFTING THE PATIENT

This can present multiple challenges. Note the pictures and comments on how to lift without injuring yourself. You must get into shape to care for dementia patients so you should work out as often as possible with walking, weights, and stretches. Ask your PCP to write a script for a Hoyer Lift, which will assist you in lifting the patient. You do not want to injure yourself because there is no one else to care for your patient if you are incapacitated. If you require 911 assistance for lifting your patient, please call and ask for *lift assist* from the 911 operator. There is no charge for *lift assist*. If they send an ambulance, the charges are substantial. Again, record *details* about all you do for your patient.

How to sit someone up who is lying in bed:

1. Position yourself at the side of the bed. Keep your feet shoulder-width apart and knees bent.

2. Place one of your arms under their legs and the other under their back.

3. Slide their legs over to the edge of the bed while you lift the top part of their body to a sitting position, holding the person close to you because it is better on your back.

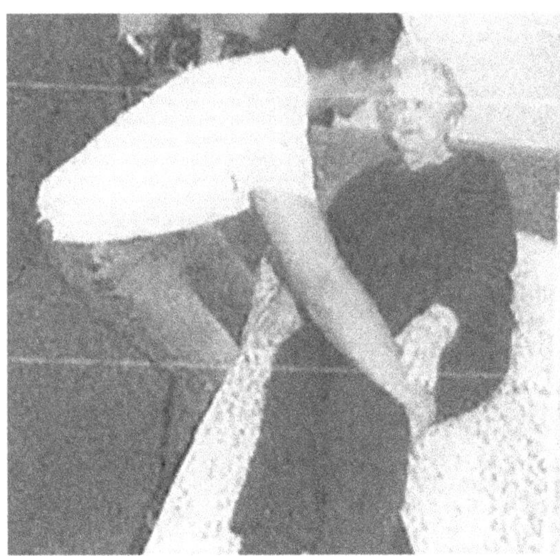
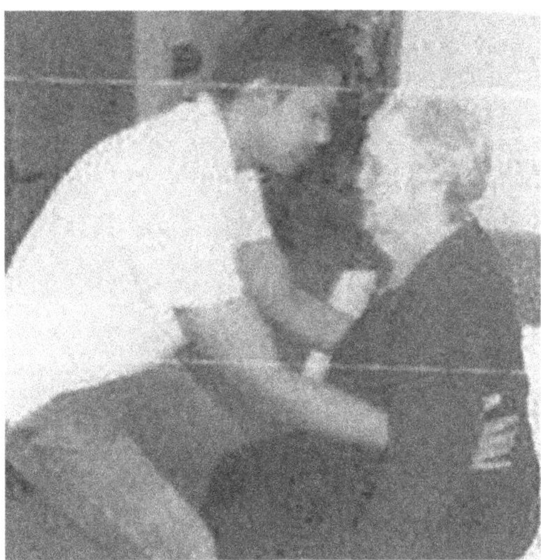

How to help someone go from sitting to standing:

1. Stand in front of them with your feet shoulder-width apart and your knees slightly bent. Do not bend your back.

2. Have the person place their feet flat on the floor, slightly apart.

3. Ask the person to place their hands around your arms, while you place your arms around their back and clasp your hands together. If you have a lifting belt, place it around the person's waist and grasp the belt when lifting the person.

4. Lift the person from the seated position, hold them close to you, leaning back slightly and shifting your feet if necessary.

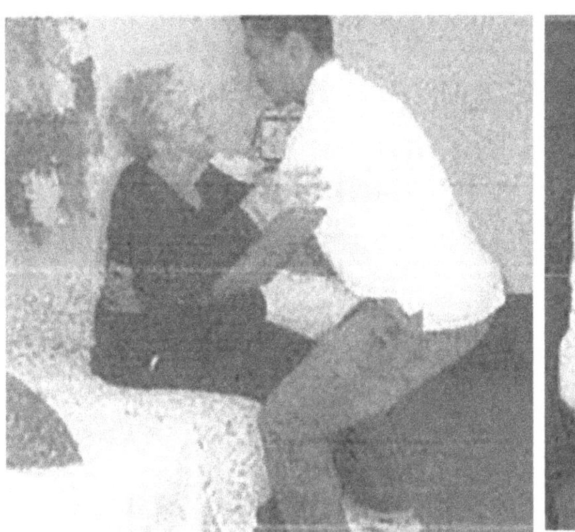 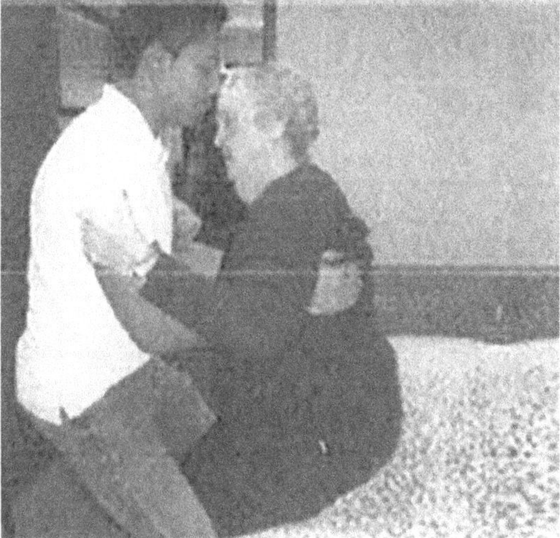

How to help someone sit down safely from a standing position:

As Alzheimer's disease progresses, actions as simple as sitting in a chair can become difficult. When this happens to the person you are caring for, try to guide them to the chair and show them how to sit down. If they still have trouble, or are unsteady on their feet:

1. Position your arms around their trunk while they are standing.

2. Have them place their hands on your upper arms.

3. Pivot or walk them until the back of their knees touches the chair.

4. Then bend your knees and lower the person into the chair. Keep your back straight and do not twist at the waist. If the chair has armrests, have the person place each hand on the corresponding armrest before you lower them, to help with stability.

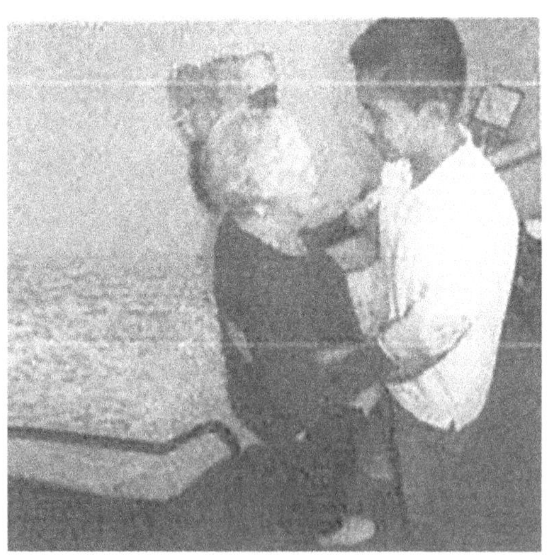
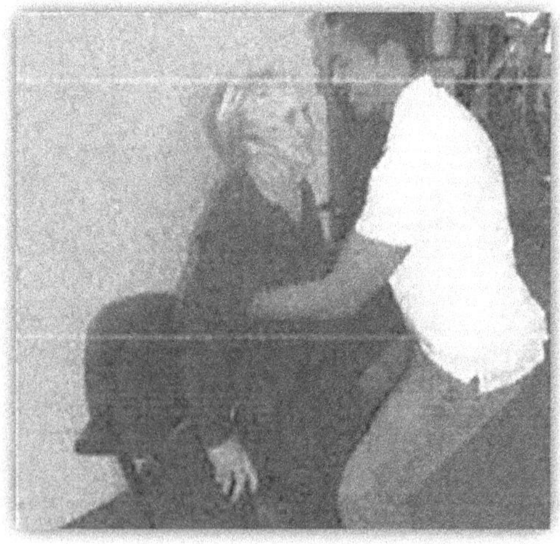

TAKING CARE OF
THE CAREGIVER

Taking care of the caregiver means just that, taking care of yourself. You may think you can do it all with no problems! But after three days of little sleep and worrying, you will become exhausted. You may need immediate help. Remember the family meeting you had? Put those people to work *now*. Also, look to outside sources for help. You need to begin the process of bringing people into your home to assist you.

Organizations like *Visiting Angels* and *Comfort Keepers* are just a few that can begin the process. If your patient has trouble with your bringing in people, use the excuse that these strangers are there to help you clean and manage the household chores. Make up a story; it's no longer a lie. You are protecting your loved one and yourself.

Let the people know that you will give them a duster to look like they are cleaning and ask them every once in a while to dust something even though their primary purpose is to watch and talk to the patient. Make sure that they go along with your request. It is not their job to correct the patient or to explain the real reason for their presence. You might begin the process of locating a private person or agency for people to care for your loved one with a conversation with your hairdresser or the director of libraries in your area. These folks know almost everything and everybody and can usually give you names and numbers of folks that are available to help. This help will give you time to shop, take a nap, and exercise.

You will begin to organize activities into fifteen-to-twenty-minute blocks. You are putting yourself on a regimen to accomplish all your task in the allotted time while help is on site. Shopping as recreation will no longer exist for you. You will have a list of what you need, and you will begin buying only what is on the list and moving on to the next task. You are actually "buying time." You may need a thirty-minute nap; take it because other chores are awaiting completion, and you have to be up for the tasks at hand. Exercise, walk, jog, lift weights, take stretches, or ride a bike—you now need to get in shape to help care for your patient/loved one. Engage in some type of exercise and diversionary activity every day because this helps you physically and mentally to get you through the day. Think *only one day at a time.* Plan for one day only. If you are thinking long-term, that would be "dinner tonight" (my sense of humor).

Put yourself on a schedule. Wake up two hours before you wake up your patient. This gives you time to go through your personal routine, eat breakfast, and plan your day.

PATIENT ROUTINE

You will begin to establish a daily routine for your patient so that he or she becomes comfortable with all that is going on. This process takes about ten to fourteen days before it becomes effective, so you will need patience in programming them to certain times and corresponding activities.

1. Good sleep hygiene (seven to eight hours of sleep), quality of sleep impacts thinking the next day and longer.
2. Have a clear schedule and structure in a daily routine.
3. Learn/teach new skills (painting, pottery, knitting).
4. Cognitive exercises (keep a daily journal, puzzles, drawing etc.).

5. Physical exercise and training help decrease risk of falls, slows down disease progressions and minimizes future hospitalizations (thirty minutes and four days a week).

6. Yoga, meditation, Tai Chi, physical therapy, speech therapy provides social engagement as well as cognitive health.

7. Heart healthy diet (Mediterranean diet).

8. Decrease alcohol intake to minimize falls and confusion.

9. People with yearly goals can bounce back better from medical setbacks, so work with your family to agree on goals your loved one could look forward to.

10. Keep an eye out for anxiety and depression and discuss pros and con treatments with your health care provider. Anxiety/depression decreases social engagement and the quality of life for your loved one.

For example, wake them up at 8:30 a.m. every day and say the same thing to them every day. "It's 8:30 a.m., and your wife/ girlfriend/ husband/boyfriend is here to greet you."

(Remember the comment earlier about listening to the patient and knowing where they are in their thinking?) That is why you need to be the correct person waking them. Wear the same clothes to do the task. Plan to buy duplicates of the same outfits so that you can maintain consistency. Tell them the time and date and begin their spa time (or whatever you want to call the bathroom routine). Serve *breakfast* at 10:00 a.m. with the same food such as two fried eggs, toast, coffee, and orange juice. Whatever you prepare will become their breakfast every day.

Serve *lunch* between 1:00 p.m. and 1:30 p.m. such as a sandwich of some kind, fruit, water, and a cookie or chocolate treat. Make sure they drink the water in order to remain hydrated throughout the day. They may also color pictures or put puzzles together with your help or the person you brought in for help.

Make sure there are daily activities including exercises for the patient. If the patient can walk outside, go along for the walk. Having soft background music on a stereo, radio, or cell phone will also help the calming process. Keep the patient comfortable but still occupied with activities.

Have the patient nap at around 3:30 p.m. or 4:00 p.m. with a 5:00 p.m. wake up by you with an invitation to a "patio party" or "cocktails in the family room." Make waking up from a nap an event. You might both enjoy the party. Once the patient awakes, freshen them up with a little cologne. Comb their hair, wash their hands, and change them if needed. Then move on to the "party."

Dinner will be served always at 6:00 p.m. Say, "Please join me for dinner." Note that I did not give them options on the party or dinner. I just told them what they were going to do. Move the patient to the dinner table, and when you serve dinner, make sure their plate of food is cut up before serving it. Do not cut up the food in front of them because that may seem very degrading!

You will need to monitor the temperature of everything that is served to the patient, making sure it is not too hot or too cold. Use your finger to make sure that the temperature is good. Again, do not monitor temperature in front of the patient. The period directly after dinner could be "movie time." You may wish to try using Netflix or a movie that they enjoy from your disc or tape collection. You may be watching it for the twentieth time, but if it is a favorite film, then watch it yet again. This may give you a break to read something you enjoy.

After the movie (or about 9:00 p.m.), it should be around *bedtime*, so off to bed you go with the patient. Create a *routine* here also. Give the patient his or her evening medications making sure the pills are ingested. Brush their teeth, dress them for bed and, with a hug, tuck the patient in.

If you can get a long sleeve nightshirt on them, this becomes comfortable for them, but you can also use the underarm fabric to help them out of bed in the morning. If you pull their arms or hands, you can risk injuring them, and they may be unable to let you know that you are hurting them.

The long-sleeved shirt solves two purposes: keeping them warm and using the clothing to get them up in the morning (note the lift picture in the previous page). If someone comes in to relieve you, they must also keep the schedule each day. You may need to write the plan down for others. If you or others change the routine, you will need to *start all over again*! Going back to square one is seldom any fun for anyone! "Back to square one is no fun!"

CAR, OUCH!

Driving provides many people with a sense of freedom and mobility. However, a person with dementia must not be driving. However, taking away the keys and the car is not easy. You most likely will need to become their personal chauffer. Tell them, "I will be driving you wherever you want or need to go whenever you want all of the time! I will be your chauffer from now on."

Remove their keys (but do not let them see you doing this). If the car that they drive is parked in the garage, move it to another place and leave the spot where their car was parked vacant. When they go to the garage and see the spot is vacant, let them know the car is in for service, and it should be back soon. You may wish to ask a friend to allow you to access a space in their garage in order to hide the car for a while.

However, *do not* tell them that "they can no longer drive." Remember: it should be, "I am your personal chauffer, and I will take you anywhere you want to go. Let's go for a ride with me in my car right now."

Take them for a ride to wherever you feel like going. Again, you are not allowing them to decide on anything other than getting in the car with you for a ride. Be very patient with them and speak softly because this conversation can easily get out of hand. No matter what they say about you (including making negative comments or even calling you names), remember that it is the disease that is talking and not your loved one. Do not take it personally!

Continue down the path of "soft conversation" and redirect them back into the house for another event if this conversation gets out of hand. But *do not* let the medical people invalidate their license. Do not give it up to anyone since they may need it in the future for identification or travel plans. Their driver's license may still be a source of pride with some patients.

They shouldn't be driving, but having an active license is *okay*. The medical people will inform the state that your patient has dementia and can no longer drive. The state will inform your insurance company, and your patient will *no longer be insured in case of an accident.*

That will most likely be indicated in fine print on your insurance policy. If someone is injured, you could be found personally liable for their costs and expenses, and in this event, if there are lawsuits, you could lose all your assets. This is not worth the gamble.

Do Not Let Your Patient Drive

In most locales, there are senior services available that can provide seniors with transportation such as Uber and Lyft. (In Allegheny County, seniors may use *access* for trips to the doctor or the grocery store, but these are unchaperoned trips and services.) But if you have only one car, the situation may change considerably.

You may need to play the chauffer role with authority. Once again, tell them something like "I'm your new chauffeur," or "I'm your new driver. I'm confident you will enjoy being chauffeured around; think how important you will feel having your own driver."

It may not be easy for many seniors to accept a change like this. But if they still have their driver's license, at least, there is some self-reliant status remaining for them. Remember, feelings are important during this journey. Hugs work well here. I wish you well on this challenge. Remember, I mentioned you need to become an actor; you are on stage to perform on being a chauffeur for you patient.

SELECTING PHYSICIANS

You really need to make good choices in selecting physicians. Begin the process with a conversation with your PCP or family doctor and get their recommendations for a neurologist. You need to research their suggestions on your computer or begin making calls to interview the doctors that were suggested.

Try to get a phone interview with the doctor that you believe will work the best with your patient. You may end up speaking with an assistant at some level, but you can at least get some feeling about their type of practice. But have your questions written and ready so you can begin the interview quickly.

Some useful questions may include the following:

- "How long have you been working with dementia patients?"
- "How do you diagnose what type of dementia patients have?"
- "What is the size of your staff to support my patient when I need answers in a timely manner?
- Who is routinely on call?"
- "What hospitals support your practice?"
- "Can we have virtual and in-person visits in a timely manner?"
- "Tell me the best reasons for me to consider using your practice?"

Once you have a physician whom you are seeing on a regular basis, the following points may be helpful:

- Tell them the list of meds your person is taking so they can better understand where you are so far in the process.

- When meds are prescribed, please make sure the doctor explains what each medication does *to* and *for* the patient.

- We want to make sure the patient is responding to the meds instead of reacting to them. We want positive results and not negative results.

- Give them a list of the changes you had noticed in the patient in the last month or longer; this is why you need to take notes. Give the doctor the time frame. Remember to *date* all your information.

Remember, once you commit to the doctor, you want to go all in on what he/she is recommending for your patient. When the doctor begins to run the show medically, you will be implementing their efforts to make your patient as comfortable as possible. I selected the Cleveland Clinic and Dr. Jagan Pillai MD, PhD. He and his staff had been most helpful in working with my wife, my daughter, and me during her FTD process.

They gave me an edge in caring for her because they were able to give me details on what was happening to her brain, what it was beginning to cause in her movement, and what part of the brain was still able to function with some normalcy. This facility and patient services were outstanding both profession- ally and personally. I can never thank them enough for their outstanding care.

When you have an MRI and CAT scan, blood draw, and spinal tap reports, ask the doctor to bring this up on his com- puter to show you where the damage is accruing in the brain and what part of the brain is affected. This can assist you in the kind of treatment you begin to deliver to your patient. Remember, you are no longer the spouse or child of the patient. You are "the caregiver."

In the beginning, I mentioned the nine different types of dementia. They are all treated differently and *treated per the spe- cific patient.* But not all the same types of dementia are treated the same way. That truly is patient-dependent. This is why I continue to make comments about paying attention to their patient's actions and comments to arrive at the best treatment for them. This person is different from the one you have been around for all those many years. You cannot categorize them from their past. He or she is a *new* and *different person,* and you need to deal with this new person on that new person's terms and how to make them at ease and comfortable.

Patients often become aggressive because they are frustrated that people are not talking to them in a manner that they understand. This is why I suggest listening to all of their comments and determining where they may be in their current thinking.

Dementia affects different parts of the brain differently, and this is why you want the doctor to be able to analyze the type of dementia and what part of the brain it is affecting. Being assertive on this issue is most important for you and the patient. *Do not* allow the medical team to talk you out of this approach just because the doctor says he uses a different process. This is what you want, and this is what you expect from the doctor. Yes, you have become demanding and rightly so!

Notes:

FOOD AND NUTRITION

Meal planning should occur in at least three to four days increments. Breakfast and lunch ideas were covered in the previous section, but now comes dinner. Cook food that is easy to swallow and easy to prepare. Vegetables should be overcooked so they are soft enough to prevent choking. Salad needs to be chopped up into small pieces in order to be swallowed easily. Cut up the meats into small pieces so the patient can chew and swallow easily. Mashed potatoes usually work well versus other types of potatoes. If you serve baked potatoes, you may need to remove the potato from the skin and mash it on their plate before serving. Remember, do not cut up their food in front of them, it is degrading. Pasta works well also, but you do need to cut it up so it is easy to pick up with a fork or spoon.

Make sure that you are serving them the foods that help them with the correct elements for good health. Their body still needs to be strong for movements in daily life. If this is difficult, talk to your PCP about a nutritionist that can put you on the right path for the correct food groups that your patient requires. *Do not be embarrassed asking for help.*

Your patient may not be able to tell you they are choking, so you need to be with them when eating so as to pay attention to their every move. If they start to choke, you will need to exercise the *Heimlich maneuver.*

How to Perform the Heimlich Maneuver

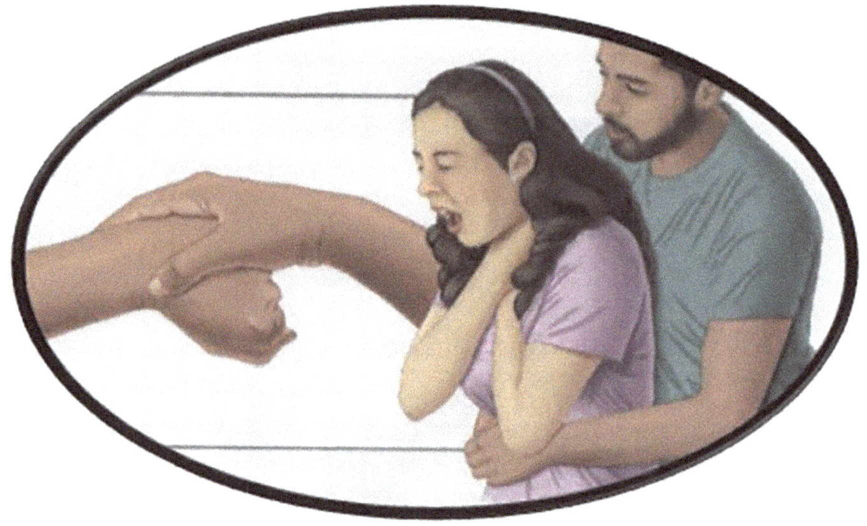

1. Stand behind the person and place your arms around their abdomen.

2. Make a fist with one hand and clasp your other hand tightly around it.

3. Place the thumb side of your fist just below their rib cage and about two inches above their belly button.

4. Sharply and quickly thrust your hands inward and upward five times.

5. Repeat this process until the object becomes freed or the person becomes unconscious. If the person becomes unconscious, start CPR.

If *you* yourself begin to choke and there is no one to help you, keep your head about you and look for a chair with a high back. From the back of the chair, lean over sharply to force the air in your lungs to push the food out of your throat and stop the choking. Another method is to lay on the floor on your arms and knees and drop your body to the floor to push the air out of your lungs and the food out of your throat. Do not be afraid to try these methods before you need them to see and experience the feeling and results. Try this a few times to make sure you have this process down in case you need to do it.

How to Perform the Heimlich Maneuver on Yourself

If you are choking, keep your head about you and follow these steps.

1. Make a fist with one hand and clasp your other hand around it.
2. Place the thumb side of your fist just below your rib cage and about two inches above your belly button.
3. Sharply and quickly thrust your hands inward and upward five times.
4. Repeat this process until the object is freed.
5. You can also try leaning over a railing or high-back chair and sharply thrust your upper abdominal area against the edge to have the object removed.

Notes:

RULES OF CONVERSATION

There are rules for you and your guest to follow in conversation with your patient. These include the following:

- Agree—never argue

- Divert—never reason

- Distract—never shame

- Reassure—never lecture

- Reminisce—never say remember

- Repeat—never say I told you

- Do what they can but never say can't

- Ask—never demand

- Encourage—never condescend

- Reinforce—never force

Every morning, in waking them up, tell them who you are: their girlfriend/wife/boyfriend/husband or whoever they think you are at that time! You are just reinforcing who you are to reassure the patient and make him or her feel more comfortable.

Give the time, date, and year, making it sound important by using voice inflections calmly. Remember, you are the beginning of their day, and you want them to be happy and pleasant all day long. Begin each day on the right note. Rehearse your waking presentation in front of a mirror. You are selling this information to your patient, and you want this to be the best beginning of their day. Remember, I said earlier you are becoming an actor, and this is how it's done. Use terms like "Good morning, Sweetie," or "It's your favorite (whatever you are to them)." Say something like "It's sunny outside, so let's begin our day today by being happy!" You also need to be smiling the entire time. Facial expressions are *very* important, and your patient reads expressions very well.

Never approach the patient you are talking to from the side or the back…only from the front. Remain at eye level and always speak softly. Never speak loudly no matter what. This may be hard to do, but I know you have to be that "actor."

Problem Solving

Solve the problem without correcting your patient and then move on. They have no idea they caused the problem. Always speak to them in soft tones and face-to-face so they will respond positively.

Also make sure visitors and other caregivers do the same with your patient. You are acting again, and you need to be the actor on stage all day long. Explain this to outside caregivers and note when (as below).

Caregiver A _______________ Date__________

Caregiver B_______________ Date__________

Make sure you inform all guests, family members, and friends about how to speak to your patient. You must make sure they *never* ask the question, "Do you know who I am?" If they did know who you are, they would most likely greet you by saying your name. But they sometimes may not remember who you are, let alone people that only show up occasionally.

Try to help guests, family, and friends by telling them how best to speak with your patient. They may say, "Hey, I've known your mom for thirty years, and I know how to speak to her." Be assertive in letting these people know that this is not the same person they have known for thirty years. Please have guests tell the patient their name and that they are here to visit. Have them tell the patient about their trip to your house or about their day so far and have them do most of the talking. Your patient will probably listen intently and may say something that is not relevant, but just move the conversation along. It really does not matter.

Let the people visiting know that they need to do the talking and storytelling about old times if that is important to the visit. Make sure that the guest does not quiz them on their conversation by saying, "Tell me what I just said?" You need to remain nearby during these conversations so they do not get out of hand.

Make sure that the guest does not correct your patient. No matter what is said, just move on in the conversation. You most likely will feel a bit tired after visits from family and friends. But remember to work at keeping your patient on the timetable that you have established. Very few people know how to converse with dementia patients, and you are the teacher for your patient. You also need to be patient with your guests; some of them have never had this experience, and you may need to guide them.

All phone calls need to be monitored. You do not want your loved one to be giving away your money to callers asking for donations. This happens a lot more often than you may suspect. Calls from friends are just as important. They may ask your patient, "How are you doing?" and "What will you be doing?" Your patient may say, "I'm having Mom over for dinner tonight," and the friend may respond by saying, "Don't you remember that your mom died ten years ago, and you were at the funeral? Don't you remember I was with you at that time?"

This is where you need to be assertive and monitor the calls. Your patient will become more upset, and the rest of the day is going to be difficult for both of you because of this conversation. When you begin to hear this type of questioning, ask the person on the other side of the phone to please not correct your patient.

Terminate the conversation perhaps by saying something like "We need to have her go for testing now." It may not be true, but it's an easy way to end the call, save face, and move on. This happens a lot more than you may think, and you will be helping your patient by not ruining their day or yours.

On a different note, if your patient brings up his or her mother, this may tell you that he or she may be living in a time period over ten years ago. This may provide you with a time frame in which to be speaking with them in an area they can understand.

This will probably be most appreciated because they may be better able to relate and feel they are fully involved in the conversation. But when they are corrected on times, dates, and events, their frustration may carry over for the remainder of the day. The rest of the day then becomes more challenging for you and them. These are some of the issues that may cause your patient to be frustrated or angry and may take out their frustration on you. But remember that this is not the same person you have known for all these years. You are dealing with a new person and trying to work around what the new person had become.

Have patience!

Notes:

HUMOR AS A TOOL

Humor is essential in dealing with a dementia patient. Laugh out loud; you will need humor to take both of you through the day. And don't be afraid to repeat yesterday's joke! Your patient most likely does not remember it, so you get to tell it again.

Besides, after repeating the same joke over and over, you tend to become very good at telling jokes. You will become impressed at your improved delivery of the jokes.

Humor from the internet or your phone can help you to find new jokes. If you have not been good at joke telling, write down a word or two that helps you remember the joke. It's worth the effort. It sometimes helps both of you to laugh. Other times, just a simple play on words helps. Something like "I need patience, but I'm not a doctor, so I have no patients." I believe you get the hint of the word play.

Start making fun of your new activities…

"I'm becoming your new personal chef, Garson. We are having ________ for dinner tonight!"

"I am your new social director. Let's get started and tour the house. Show me the pictures that are on the walls and tell me something about them." They may say something or just stare at the picture, and you can make something up about the picture and then move on to the next picture.

"I am your new doctor's assistant. Time to take your blood pressure," etc.

Write things down so you can refer to them as time permits. Let people that are caring for your patient use some of these tactics about touring the house and reviewing pictures or plants or vases. Picture books of past events are also great, but remember where your patient is in their time frame of thinking. Some picture books may not be appropriate, so move those picture books to another place! The idea is to keep your patient active.

Reassure him or her that "I am your personal driver" whenever you can slip that into the conversation. It may keep that relationship in their mind, and hopefully, they will always remain committed to your driving them without issues.

Notes:

FINDING SOLUTIONS TO PROBLEMS

Avoid social media! If you spend too much time on social media, you will probably have people complaining at length about their problems. It seems that everyone enhances their issues, and few people explore solutions. You need information and solutions. There are websites that give you knowledge and that may help you solve your problems! Here are a few excellent resources:

- *www.alz.pa.com* for Pennsylvania residence but I'm sure your state has the same site using your state abbreviations. It's free.

- *www.arden-coiurt.org* is another outstanding website that has Dr. Tam Cummings as the teacher, and they have a presentation the first Thursday of every month at

11:00 a.m.; it is outstanding and will help you in your challenges. It's *free*. View their website to look up old presentations that you need the information from to help you with a specific problem. You may also call these people that are most helpful.

- An organization that is truly great for dementia patients and dementia facilities is *www.aging.pa.gov/aging-services*. This is another website you may need to put your state abbreviations in for Pennsylvania, and I'm sure they will have similar information.

SUPPORT GROUPS

If you are intimidated by computers, you may be able to call your local or state medical association or a health-care association to find a group that supports dementia in your area. It may be quite worthwhile to consider joining such a group.

When a health-care organization runs the support group, they usually have a professional on staff at the meetings and can provide you with ideas and other local information that is professional and helpful.

People in these groups may be currently having the same problems as you, or they may have experienced similar problems in the past and may be able to help suggest a solution for you.

These groups can both be very useful and may also create some friendships at the same time. They could also have the names of doctors who are very good with dementia patients.

Your church may also have similar groups that may be very helpful. You don't necessarily have to attend every meeting, but it can give you some support in caring for your loved one. You most likely will learn that you are not alone in your challenge with your patient and that help is all around you. If so, you should consider taking advantage of this help; most of the time, it is provided for free.

But take *notes* at these support group meetings. While it may give you a break from your caregiving, it can also give you invaluable knowledge and information on how to care for your loved one.

And prayers help no matter what your personal belief system may be. Pray to your God for wisdom and knowledge in helping you to care for your patient. You most likely cannot do it alone, and I'm sure HE will grant you the wisdom, knowledge, patience, and strength necessary to care for your loved one. Pray to Him for divine help as you perform your new job of caregiving. You very likely will need all the help you can muster, and special help from above is especially worth the effort.

Notes:

HEALTH-CARE AGENCY

Selecting the proper agency to help you in providing care for your patient is a critical and an arduous task. You may find an agency that will work with you in the very beginning, as I mentioned earlier. Organizations such as Visiting Angels or Comfort Keepers are excellent resources. But once your patient needs more than they can provide, you need help to find home care agencies that can send qualified people who possess the specific experience and education necessary to care for dementia patients.

You may discover an agency that can work with you when attending a support group meeting. Explore all options, and then select the agency that best meets your needs and times for caring. You must make sure that they keep your patient on the same schedule that you are establishing with *no* deviations.

Write the schedule down for the home caregivers so that there is no mistake as to what needs to be done and when to do it.

But if you are using different terms for activities, make sure the home caregivers use the same language. I used "art class" for coloring pictures and "PE class" for doing exercise. My wife was an educator, and using those terms made sense to her. At least that was what I believed, and it did not seem degrading. These agency personnel are taking your place for a short time, and you may want your patient to feel there is no difference, whether it is you or home care givers to which they are speaking. *Consistency* is the key!

I used St. Barnabas, a local organization, for their home care service. Their caregivers were very professional and personal with my wife. The care they extended matched my established schedule and routines, and we saw no deviations. They were outstanding.

Notes:

RESTAURANTS

If you are still able to dine out, plan to always call ahead to the restaurant and explain your situation. For example, you will need a table in a corner with your patient's back to the wall so that they may see everyone moving around in front of them. Let the person that answered the phone know if the patient tends to blurt out verbiage or is unable to speak so that the server understands the situation ahead of time.

But you do not want to have that conversation with the server in front of your patient! That could prove to be degrading!

Explain up front that the food needs to be cut up in the kitchen and that the vegetables need to be a little overcooked. Make sure the side dishes served do not have garnishes or decorative items that are not to be eaten.

If you need a special drink, you may have to bring the items for that drink to the restaurant. They very likely *do not* have every possible ingredient for every possible drink.

Try dining at about the same time that you would normally be dining at home. Again, consistency is the key!

The environment within the restaurant may also prove to be a nice change of pace for both you and your patient. You may have a nice evening out, and that becomes enjoyable. The Alzheimer's organization has a card that is shown below. It is available for free and is very helpful for you and the people taking care of you in the restaurant. It also works very well for travel, especially with TSA.

alzheimer's association®
Greater Pennsylvania Chapter

Information, Referral, Education and Care
We're here to help and offer hope. All day. Every day.

Helpline 1.800.272.3900

alz.org/pa   fb.com/alzgpa   @alzgpa

PLEASE BE PATIENT...

The person with me has Dementia/Alzheimer's disease and has forgotten how to act in certain situations.

Thank you for understanding.

Alzheimer card picture

TRAVEL

If you can still travel, please be prepared to spend extra time in every situation, from bathrooms to TSA and from ticket counter to boarding, along with inflight service. Tell the flight attendant the situation (show them the card above so they understand) and plan from there in seating both of you.

When landing, you may need to pay extra attention because you do not want the patient wandering off in an unfamiliar airport environment. This could prove disastrous!

Have your plan put together with the people you are meeting before you begin the journey. If they can meet you at the arrival gate, so much the better. If that is not always the case, you need to consider every possible situation before you embark on your trip. *Details.*

If you are driving to your destination, your problems are a little less trying since patients are comfortable in the car that is familiar to them. But when you stop for fuel again, pay attention! You don't want them wandering around a service plaza without supervision. Issues can happen, and you need to anticipate all the challenges that may take place.

Remember, you are taking the person out of their structured environment, and this will truly challenge you. I'm sure you thought I purchased tickets or reservations six months ago because they were so cheap for the event or trip, and now the person is six more months into the disease and are becoming more challenging. If you think this is becoming an issue, *cancel the trip!* It is not worth the stress on you for this adventure. You need to make sure that patients are capable of traveling before you go down this path.

Notes:

PLACEMENT IN A CAREGIVING FACILITY

When all else fails and you are unable to care for your loved one, it becomes your decision alone to place them in a care facility. Begin by interviewing dementia facilities. Here are some things to look for:

- The caregiver to patient ratio
- Safety
- Doctor on staff or on call
- Size and cleanliness of facility
- Verbal environment
- Size of patient rooms and type of furnishings
- Activities during the day (observe)

Go to the facility several times—early, midday, and late day—so you get to see what transpires when you don't have an appointment. The staff may tell you one thing or another, but your eyes also see what is going on during these surprise visits.

You know you can expect to be paying between $9,000 and $14,000 per month plus laundry and the dispensing of medication charges. This is an expensive decision!

I mentioned Arden Court previously, and dementia is their specialty. From my observations, they do an excellent job. Other areas have the equivalent of this facility. Get recommendations from a similar agency or a support group.

I did not have to place my wife in a facility. We made the "entire journey" at home. This was a very challenging time, but I'm proud to say that I promised her I would keep her at home. I am proud to report that I was able to keep my promise.

Notes:

THE END IS COMING

Get prepared for the eventual funeral. Do not make emotional preparations in the final hours; emotions will not help you make the right decisions.

Funeral directors can take a lot of stress off your back. They do this for a living every day and understand the real issues. Give them a budget number that you can easily afford, and remember that you do not need to pay anything up front. If they ask for money up front, *leave* immediately and look for another funeral director.

Plan for flowers, services, and the obituary in the newspaper. The newspaper listing is expensive, so add those numbers to your budget. Death certificates are about $20 each, but you will need several of them for insurance and financial companies and the bank for closing accounts. Coordinate that with your financial advisor who can assist you with information for the final process. Your funeral director can assist you with the listing. Write the obituary and have someone proof and correct it.

If someone else volunteers to write one, make sure *you* read it for accuracy before it is published. Remember that while friends and relatives are going to read it so may con artists, and you could expose yourself to problems. Have a friend available to be at your house during the funeral times that are posted in the newspaper. You never know!

When death does occur, make a list of personal friends and relatives that *you* want to call. This is a sad and emotional time, so make the message short and to the point. Have a short script ready; for example, "(Name) passed away today from his or her battle with dementia. Services will be at XYZ Funeral Home (list days and times). I wanted to let you to know personally."

They will most likely offer you condolences. Accept them graciously but briefly and bid them goodbye. Then move on to each remaining name on the list.

Keep your wits about you during and after the funeral services. Remember that con artists often prey on grieving people. Get comfortable with what you want to say to explain the death of your loved one.

Explain that (name) died (or passed away, or passed, or graduated to the next dimension or transitioned to eternal life). It's your choice, and you need to feel comfortable with the phrasing.

Do not say something like "Didn't you see the obituary? It was in the paper." Never assume that your friends, relatives, and neighbors know about the death. And you do not need to go into details. People will most likely say something like "I'm sorry to hear the news." Thank them for any condolences they offer, and everyone will become more comfortable.

Keep your comments short and to the point, and move on to other topics, as appropriate.

Now comes the hard part. You need to close everything down. Call the local police department, and let them know that the patient has passed, and there is no further need for their assistance regarding your patient with dementia. Call 911 and give them the same information but ask for the supervisor, the one you wrote down earlier in the book, to make sure your information is deleted. Please also call the various doctors involved to let them know of your patient's death.

Remember to call any and all insurance companies. If money is due from existing insurance policies, make sure they get a copy of the death certificate so they will pay you.

The details of the finality of death are just ongoing. It has taken me about fifteen months to finally finish all the changes needed with my wife's passing. Grief does get in the way, but it is the price of love, and that is normal. You need to get through the grief process. There are church committees that have support groups which can help you deal with the grieving process. However, never forget that this will take some time!

The hospice group that you used may also be able to assist you with this post-death experience of losing a loved one. But don't underestimate the power of grief in your life! For months and years, your daily life was consumed with caring for a loved one; now, your days are filled with paperwork, but soon, that too will end. The process of grief can sometimes take over your day-to-day thinking, and you need to be able to make logical decisions for yourself and your future. Prayers certainly will be able to help as you navigate this necessary process.

The information above represents much of what I experienced throughout the five years that I spent caring for my wife. I hope it helps readers with the challenges they may face in caring for their loved ones at sad times such as these!

As I said above, each patient is different, and each dementia case affects each patient differently. It's invariably a patient-specific condition. But take your time. Seek patience. And always remember that your role is incredibly important to your loved one.

Remember, invariably, you will always be their most important caregiver!

"It's your show," so become the best *actor* that you can be for your patient. Grief does get in the way, but grief is indeed the price of love.

RESOURCES

Alzheimer's Association helpline

800-272-3900

Edit: Mary Louise Ellena and David G. Young

Graphic placement: Jenna McKenney

ProMedica at Arden Court

UPMC, Dr. John Wisneski

Cleveland Clinic, Dr. Jagan Pillai, https://pages.clevelandclinic.

org